CALCIUM: The Facts

Get maximum benefits from
FOSSILIZED CORAL
and important cofactors

A Health Learning Handbook
Beth M. Ley, Ph.D.

BL Publications
Detroit Lakes, MN

Copyright © 2001 by BL Publications
All rights reserved. No part of this book may be reproduced or transmitted by any means, electronic or mechanical, without written permission from the publisher:

BL Publications, Detroit Lakes, MN
For orders call 1-877-BOOKS11
email: blpub@tekstar.com

Library of Congress Cataloging-in-Publication Data
Ley, Beth M., 1964-
  Calcium : the facts : get maximum benefits from fossilized coral and important cofactors a health learning handbook / Beth M. Ley.
       p. cm. -- (A health learning handbook)
  Includes index.
   ISBN 1-890766-17-8
   1. Calcium in the body. 2. Calcium in human nutrition. 3. Calcium--Metabolism--Disorders. I. Title. II. Series.
   QP535.C2 L49 2001
   612.3'924--dc21
                                                    2001002115

Printed in the United States of America

This book is not intended as medical advice. Its purpose is solely educational. Please consult your healthcare professional for all health problems.

Credits

Cover Design: BL Publications
Cover Photo: Shohei Shirai
Proofreading: Deborah Brenk

"Use food as your medicine and medicine as your food." Hippocrates

Table of Contents

Introduction 5
Calcium: What You Need to Know 6
Osteoporosis 15
    Dental Health .20
Heart Health and High Blood Pressure 21
Muscles and Nerves 23
Cancer 24
    Colon Cancer .25
    Breast Cancer .26
Insomnia 26
Premenstrual Cramps 27
Kidney Stones 28
Calcium Sources 28
    Food High in Calcium 32
Fossilized Coral Calcium 32
Bibliography 42
Index 45
About the Author 46
Books from BL Publications 47

YOU NEED TO KNOW...
THE HEALTH MESSAGE

Do you not know that you are God's temple and that God's Spirit dwells in you? If anyone destroys God's temple, God will destroy him, For God's temple is holy and that temple you are. *1 Corinthians 3:16-17*

So, whether you eat or drink, or whatever you do, do all to the glory of God.
1 Corinthians 10:31

Introduction

Calcium is the most abundant mineral in the body. It primarily functions in your body to make your bones and teeth hard. The remaining is in your blood and soft tissues; it helps your nervous system work properly. Calcium is also important for our heart, thyroid, immune system, energy production and for cellular maintenance. It helps regulate heartbeat and is necessary for muscle contraction and allows blood to clot.

Calcium deficiencies are linked to a number of health problems including high blood pressure, cancers of the colon and breast, osteoporosis and atherosclerosis.

On average, our diets provide only half of the 1,000-1,500 mgs. daily calcium currently recommended by the National Institutes of Health; new government guidelines are expected to adjust this dose to 2,500 mg. To make sure you get enough calcium, a calcium supplement may be needed, but choosing one can be difficult. Hopefully, this book will clear up some of the confusion.

Many of our lifestyle choices, including high sugar intake, high protein (especially meat), excess caffeine and phosphoric acid (found in soda pop), some prescription drugs, and both the lack of exercise and its excessive practice, undermine our calcium stores.

Fossilized coral is an excellent source of usable calcium for the body. Fossilized coral actually contains over 70 different minerals and trace minerals (all which are needed by the body), and of which calcium is in the highest concentration. It has been used therapeutically since the 15th Century to promote health in Eastern cultures.

Calcium: What You Need to Know

When the subject of calcium comes up, milk inevitably is brought up. Research indicates that while the public largely believes milk and dairy products to be a primary source of dietary calcium, they may actually be an insufficient source. Even further, dairy products may even work to decrease calcium levels in the body. This may surprise many people as the dairy industry has done an excellent job of snowballing the public to believing that drinking milk is the answer to all one's calcium needs.

The Daily Value (DV) for calcium for healthy men and women is 1,000 mg. The actual amount of calcium an individual needs actually varies. Calcium needs increase with age. Women who have passed menopause need at least 1,500 mg. daily. Calcium absorption diminishes as we grow older due to a number of reasons including hormonal and digestive.

The calcium intake of adults living in the stone-age is estimated at three to five times the average calcium intake of U.S. adults living today. Long-term calcium restriction and/or insufficient Vitamin D may promote the development of bone fragility, high blood pressure, colon cancer and breast cancer in susceptible individuals. Conversely, improvement in calcium intake and Vitamin D status may help to prevent these serious health problems. (Barger-Lux)

Vegetarians who tend to consume a "less acidic" diet do not require as much calcium as meat eaters. High protein foods, such as meat, are acid-forming which requires the body to neutralize the low or acidic pH of the body's fluids. The body does this with calcium. If necessary, it will remove calcium from our bones to do this. This calcium is then excreted in the urine.

Calcium deficiencies do occur but it is not known for certain whether deficiencies are due entirely to inadequate intake, or a combination of factors which cause diminished absorption and utilization of the calcium we consume in our foods. Imbalances may be created from a variety of factors. I suspect it often is a combination of all of these things. This theory suggests that supplementation of calcium alone would not solve the problem. Studies also support this. Simply supplementing calcium **WILL NOT** solve the problem of osteoporosis.

As calcium is very important to our overall health, the body will attempt to regulate calcium levels in the blood, even if this means sacrificing bone. Because of this, laboratory blood tests will usually indicate that calcium and phosphorus levels are normal.

Calcium Facts:

- The human body contains about 1,100 grams of calcium – about 1.5% of our total body weight.

- Calcium, as the primary structural mineral in bone, is essential for skeletal health. In addition, the one percent of our body's supply not found in bone is likewise critical to the heart, muscles, nerve function and metabolic processes.

- We typically absorb only 30% of the dietary calcium we ingest.

- Certain dietary factors can reduce our calcium absorption even further: Fiber, caffeine, alcohol, a high-protein diet and oxalates (found in tea, beets and endive). Protein and diuretics increase urinary calcium excretion. Fiber and oxalates inhibit calcium absorption.

- 80% of all American women are calcium deficient.

- Men and women over age 30 require up to 67% more calcium than do 16 year olds.

- Calcium is not only essential as a bone-building nutrient, but also shows promise as one which helps control blood pressure. The Calcium Information Center reports that blood pressure can be reduced by increasing calcium intake.

- Calcium assists in the absorption of vitamins and helps with nerve, hormone and enzyme functioning.

- Some research findings reveal the most effective time to supplement calcium is nighttime. However, at this time, if you have an empty stomach, supplementing

---

Chalk, eggshells, milk and bones all get their dense white color from calcium.

We have more calcium than any other mineral in our bodies – 99% of it is found in our bone. It is vital throughout our lifetimes for strong bones and teeth.

NATIONAL INSTITUTE OF HEALTH OPTIMAL DAILY RECOMMENDED CALCIUM INTAKE	
Adults	1,000 mg.
Postmenopausal women	1,500 mg.
Adults over 65	1,500 mg.
Pregnant/Nursing women	1,200-1,500 mg.
Young adults (11-24)	1,200-1,500 mg.
Children under 11	800-1,200 mg.

betaine hydrochloride (a source of hydrochoric acid) or vinegar can assist absorption.

• Other studies report that calcium mineral supplements should be taken with food because the stomach will naturally produce hydrochloric acid at that time. The best advice may be to take your calcium supplement 2 to 3 times per day as it is believed that the body can only absorb about 500 mg. elemental calcium at a time.

• The form of the calcium taken and which co-nutrients it is taken with are important in achieving the most beneficial results from a calcium supplement. Vitamin D-3 is needed for optimal calcium absorption.

• The calcium in milk and dairy products is actually poorly absorbed. One cup of cooked broccoli actually contains more usable calcium (53% of 178 mg. = 94 mg.) than 1 oz. of cheese (32% of 220 mg. = 70 mg.)! See page 35 for more calcium absorption rates!

Broccoli (1 cup, cooked) actually contains more usable calcium than 1 oz. of cheese!

Assimilation

Calcium absorption and assimilation by the body is not always easy. The calcium we take in through foods or supplements won't do us much good if it cannot be easily digested or assimilated. Once it enters the blood stream, its value will be limited by the availability of important calcium co-factors. We cannot hope to maintain or restore strong, healthy bones without them.

Proper stomach acidity is required for calcium to dissolve. If you are not sure you have adequate stomach acidity, try taking your calcium supplement with one tablespoon vinegar mixed with one tablespoon honey or with a hydrochloric acid supplement. Sometimes it may be better to chew the tablets to help break them down.

Plant sources of calcium tend to be much easier to absorb by the body than dairy sources. Meat and dairy products are high in phosphorus and protein, which are detrimental to calcium levels in the body. Phosphorus interferes with calcium availability and protein increases calcium excretion.

> *According to the American Heart Association, studies show that vegetarians absorb and retain more calcium from foods than do nonvegetarians.*

Calcium Co-factors

In order to absorb and assimilate calcium (and other important minerals) for good bone health, Vitamins A, D and C, and magnesium are necessary. A diet too high in cholesterol makes it difficult for the body to assimilate the fat-soluble Vitamins A and D.

Vitamin D mineralizes the skeleton by elevating calcium and phosphorus in the blood. It works with the parathyroid hormone to stimulate absorption in the intestinal tract and to increase renal reabsorption of calcium in the distal tubules. (Yamamoto)

As we grow older, our ability to produce Vitamin D diminishes. (Tanaka) Vitamin D-3 supplementation (4,000 IU daily) aids postmenopausal women with osteoporosis. (Christianson, Ott) Larger amounts (7,500 IU daily) have shown better results, but may also be associated with the increased risk of hypercalcemia (elevated calcium levels) and possible kidney stones. (Aloia)

Magnesium is very important for calcium to be used by the body, and especially the bones as it acts like a gate keeper.

Note: Supplementing the hormone pregnenolone is a safe precursor to testosterone, progesterone and the estrogens, 50-100 mg. daily.

Why Dairy Products Are a Poor Source of Calcium

1. *Dairy products are high in protein which increases calcium excretion from the bones and body.*

2. *Dairy products are high in phosphorus which inhibits calcium absorption.*

3. *Dairy products are very low in magnesium which is needed for bone to use the calcium which is absorbed.*

4. *Dairy products may contain saturated fat which makes calcium absorption more difficult.*

Mineral Balancing

One of the basic principles of nutrition is that no nutrient ever works alone. Calcium is by no means an exception to this rule. Calcium needs to be balanced with other minerals according the the ratios as they are present in the body.

Mineral imbalances are the underlying cause of many of our health troubles. The body contains over 70 minerals. Genesis 2:7 tells us, *And the LORD God formed man of the dust of the ground, and breathed into his nostrils the breath of life; and man became a living soul.* The mineral content of the "dust" of the earth is reflected in sea water, which contains 84 of the 103 elements in the Periodic Table of Elements.

All nutrients in the body, especially the minerals, operate in a biochemical symphony. It is the combination of these elements (in the correct proportions) that allows the body to function harmoniously. If there is a lack of or abundance of any particular substance, problems result.

For example, the four main minerals in the body, calcium, magnesium, sodium and potassium, regulate two areas of critical importance in the body, the thyroid and adrenal glands. If these four minerals are at normal levels, and everything else is in balance, these glands can function optimally.

Imbalances will cause either overactivity which can result in stress or underactivity which results in low energy levels and insufficiency. Calcium and potassium regulate the activity of the thyroid gland. If the ratio between them and the mineral levels is normal, the thyroid functions at maximum energy levels.

Calcium slows down the activity of the thyroid, and potassium speeds it up. If the level of calcium is too high, the energy level of the thyroid will be slowed down. If the level of potassium is too high, the thyroid will be overactive and will eventually wear out completely because of too much stress.

If one mineral level is too high or too low, it affects all other minerals in the body. No mineral works alone. For example, some people take an iron supplement because they are tired. This is what can happen: Iron causes sodium levels to rise as a result of stimulating the adrenal glands. Magnesium levels will go down because sodium lowers magnesium. Calcium will go down because magnesium and calcium strive to be at the same level. Calcium and potassium move in opposite directions, so when calcium goes down, potassium goes up. As many as 21 minerals can be affected by altering just one. Again, no mineral works alone.

We all can benefit from an absorbable calcium/mineral formulation, especially those most vulnerable to bone loss; women during and past menopause, anyone with questionable diets or sedentary lifestyles and seniors (men included).

While osteoporosis is most commonly associated with calcium deficiencies, there are actually more than 150 diseases scientifically documented to be related to calcium deficiency. Prevention is the most economical way to approach this, as well as almost all other health problems. Following are some of the major deficiency problems: Osteoporosis, high blood pressure, pregnancy-related high blood pressure, insomnia, colon cancer, breast cancer, menstrual cramps, muscle cramps and restless-legs syndrome.

Calcium is used for much more in the body. It's also dissolved in the fluids in the body, those inside cells and those that bathe cells. There, it helps muscles spring into action and aids proper blood clotting. It assists nerves in transmitting impulses and helps launch hormones and enzymes on their journeys to inner organs.

Serum Calcium Levels Closely Guarded

Calcium levels in the blood rarely vary more than 5% above or below normal concentrations. When calcium levels fall below this, parathormone (produced by the parathyroid glands) act upon the body to withdraw calcium from other places in the body to replenish calcium levels in the blood. If calcium levels in the blood become too high, calcitonin (produced by the thyroid) lowers it. The active form of Vitamin D-3 (Cholecalciferol), acting like a hormone, also regulates calcium levels in the blood.

Calcium Enemies

Many concerned about getting adequate calcium intake in their diet, may need not be so concerned <u>if the many enemies to calcium in the body were avoided.</u> These include:

- Alcohol, caffeine and other diuretics
- Smoking
- Fiber supplements (should not be taken at the same time as calcium supplements.)
- Diet high in protein, sugar and refined carbohydrates (increases pH – calcium is used as a buffer)
- High phosphorus intake (found in meat, dairy

products and soda pop)

- Foods containing oxalates. These bind calcium, inhibiting its absorption in the body. These include (ranked from highest to lowest concentration):

Spinach	Rhubarb	Beets
Swiss chard	Wheat germ	Pecans
Peanuts	Chocolate	Tea (black)

- High sodium intake

- Saturated fat

Osteoporosis

Osteoporosis is the result of a loss of normal bone density, marked by thinning of bone tissue and the growth of small holes in the bone. Osteoporosis means "porous bone."

More than 1.5 million Americans have fractures related to osteoporosis at an annual cost in the U.S. health care system of 10 billion dollars. Complications of hip fractures are a major killer of women. In many cases, the fracture precedes a fall rather than being caused by it. Soft, spongy bone (found in the jaw, hips, spine and wrists) is the first to go.

Great pain may be experienced with osteoporosis, but fortunately it is preventable and can be aided with the help of special nutritional supplements. For those who are affected, it can be also be disfiguring and debilitating. There are no warning signs that a bone is weak enough to fracture. The only sure way of knowing your risk is by a bone density test. A DEXA scan is one of the most accurate tests available for bone density. It is painless, accurate, non-invasive and takes only a few minutes to perform. If the results indicate you have low bone density, you must take steps to stop bone loss and build new bone as soon as possible, before a weakened bone breaks.

Weakened, less dense bones are more susceptible to fractures and breakage. X-rays of osteoporotic bones often reveal many hairline fractures in areas such as the lumbar spine region, wrists, forearms, legs and hips. These fractures are not only painful, they further weaken the bone.

Bone cells, like all cells in the body, are continually renewing themselves. This process involves bone reabsorption where minerals are removed from the bones, and bone formation where minerals are put back into new bone. When bone reabsorption occurs at a faster rate than new bone is formed, the result is bone loss, medically termed *osteoporosis.*

After our third decade, the level of our bone mass plateaus. Bone loss begins in the fourth or fifth decade of life. In women, bone loss accelerates after menopause. Among men, it accelerates after age 65. Men lose bone too, although only about half as quickly as women.

Are You at Risk?

Osteoporosis is not inevitable for everyone, but there are numerous factors which increase one's susceptibility to the problem.

Women are more likely to develop osteoporosis than men because men start with a larger bone mass and do not go through the dramatic hormonal changes that women do. **Caucasian women** with northern **European** blood ties are at the highest risk.

Individuals at additional risk are those who take steroid hormones such as **anti-inflammatory agents** commonly prescribed for arthritis and joint discomfort.

Smokers, and those who consume **alcohol** or **caffeine** (coffee, tea, cola, etc.), are at a higher risk.

A diet high in **animal protein** induces a calcium deficiency.

A diet high in **saturated fat** reduces calcium absorption.

Fiber (as important as it is for good health) makes calcium more difficult to absorb if eaten at the same time.

Individuals who consume a large amount of **sweets** and **refined carbohydrates** are at a higher risk.

Individuals who experience prolonged **stress,** or live a **sedentary** life and do not get adequate exercise are at a higher risk.

Symptoms of Osteoporosis

Frequent broken bones
Loss of height
Cramps in legs and feet (often at night)
Bone pain
Lower back pain, leg pain
Fractures of the hip, wrist, spine
Dowager's hump (forward bending of the spine) and other deformities
Fatigue
Brittle or soft fingernails
Premature grey hair
Heart palpitations

Osteoporosis Facts

• During a lifetime women lose approximately 50% of the cancellous bone and 30% of cortical bone. Men lose about 30% and 20% of the same.

• The average American loses 1.5 inches of height <u>each</u> <u>decade</u> after menopause as a result of vertebral collapse. This means you may be 3 inches shorter at 70 than you were at age 50!

• Osteoporosis is the cause of 90% of all fractures after age 65.

• One out of three women over age 65 will suffer hip fracture, which is fatal in one out of every five cases.

• Osteoporosis causes 40% of all people to lose their teeth after age 60. (Periodontal disease is osteoporosis of the mouth.)

• Osteoporosis is primarily a disease of "modernized" countries. Not all areas of the world have seen the dramatic increase in the incidence of osteoporosis that we have in the U.S. This may be due to "estrogen dominance" created due to the abundant use of hormones and chemicals in our foods.

• **<u>Men are not exempt</u>**. Most of us think of osteoporosis as a woman's problem. Men are not excluded from this epidemic, statistics show that one out of every six men over 90 will fracture a hip.

• Prevention is by far the easiest and most cost effective approach to osteoporosis.

What Causes Osteoporosis?

Contrary to popular belief, osteoporosis is not due to a lack of dietary calcium. It is the result of the loss of calcium and other minerals found in bone caused by a number of factors. Some of these we have control over. Some we do not.

An upset in body chemistry results in increased susceptibility to health problems. When all the minerals, hormones, pH level and other elements are in balance, the body is in homeostasis and the body runs most efficiently. When an imbalance occurs, the body makes certain adjustments through its numerous feedback systems, designed to keep the internal body chemistry in balance.

Changes in the acid-base balance of the body are tremendous contributors to bone loss. Even a slight decrease in pH (acidosis) leads calcium loss from bone as calcium salts are needed as an alkaline buffer. Acidosis can be caused by a diet high in protein (especially red meat), phosphoric acid (found in soda pop) and sugar and other refined carbohydrates.

The body functions best when all the needed nutrients, including minerals, are present in their proper proportions. But if there is a shortage of just one mineral, the system will weaken and begin to lose efficiency. With the balance of the body off, the body cannot operate optimally and eventually disease will set in. In this case, osteoporosis.

> *Simply supplementing calcium alone WILL NOT help osteoporosis!*

Many people assume that osteoporosis results from a calcium deficiency. While this may be true in some situations, it is by by no means the only cause of osteoporosis. Mineral **imbalance**s and many other contributing factors are just as common. If other factors are causing a calcium deficiency or what appears to be a calcium deficiency, resulting in the depletion of bone, then the true cause of osteoporosis is **not** a calcium deficiency, but the other factors.

The medical establishment considers a daily supplement of 1,000-1,500 mg. elemental calcium with a Vitamin D supplement to be an adequate and inexpensive therapy for senile osteoporosis. (Praet) At least 12 intervention studies have established the skeletal benefit of increased calcium intake among women in late postmenopause. (Barger-Lux) However, the most effective form of calcium has not been closely reviewed, as well as the significance of the 70 plus other minerals in the body.

Dental Health

While total body bone loss is known as osteoporosis, bone loss in the oral cavity, resulting in less support for the teeth, is called periodontal disease. Reduction of bone mineralization due to insufficient dietary calcium and a reduction in the calcium to phosphorous ratio increases the risk for periodontal disease. Alveolar bone (referring to the upper jaw bone) which has the highest rate of renewal, is affected first and consequently, is the most severely affected in the long term. Adequate calcium intake reduces inflammation and tooth mobility in patients suffering from gingivitis and bleeding gums. (Ortega)

Heart Health and High Blood Pressure

Heart disease risk factors include at least two factors which can be reduced through calcium supplementation: hypertension and elevated cholesterol.

Proper amounts of calcium in the body help regulate dietary fats and cholesterol levels in the blood. In the intestines, calcium can combine with other nutrients and foods – such as saturated fat – to create compounds that cannot be absorbed into the body. In one study, a group of people getting approximately 1,000 mgs. of calcium a day from fortified foods and 1,000 mgs. from supplements excreted twice as much saturated fat as people getting lower amounts of calcium. They also had an 11% drop in harmful LDL cholesterol.

The causes of high blood pressure, such as above 40/90 mmHg (millimeters of mercury), are largely unknown. Diseases affecting the kidneys, adrenals or other glands can occasionally raise blood pressure, which is termed secondary high blood pressure, but most often, high blood pressure happens for unknown reasons.

Women who are overweight, have diabetes, are African-American or taking birth control pills carry the greatest risk of getting high blood pressure. High blood pressure is very common among women. According to the American Heart Association, if you are between ages 35 and 55, chances are about one in four that you have it, while nearly one out of two women over 55 have it.

Uncontrolled, high blood pressure increases your risk of heart disease, kidney failure and stroke.

Many studies have found that calcium supplements, typically 800-1,500 mg. daily, lowers blood high pressure. (Bucher) While doctors do not know the exact mechanism of calcium's action, I suspect it involves the regulation of sodium and potassium levels in the body. Interactions between dietary nutrients are critical in the effect of calcium on blood pressure, particularly sodium and potassium. (McCarron)

Data from both epidemiologic surveys and clinical trials show that calcium metabolism is altered in individuals with hypertension, indicating a primary role of calcium in the etiology, prevention and treatment of hypertension. (McCarron)

Magnesium, typically 350-500 mg. per day, and potassium can also help lower blood pressure. The results are particularly effective in people who are taking "depleting diuretic" medications. (Dyckner)

Pregnancy-related High Blood Pressure

Calcium also plays a role in the etiology, prevention and treatment of pregnancy-induced hypertension (PIH). The precise factors involved in its cause are unclear, but several alterations in calcium metabolism have been identified suggesting an inverse correlation between dietary calcium intake and incidence of PIH. Evidence suggests a possible beneficial effect of supplemental calcium for pregnant women, especially teens. (Ritchie)

Calcium supplementation during pregnancy can increase the intake in those with a deficiency or can provide a pharmacologic effect in individuals with an adequate calcium intake. A systematic review examined randomized, double-blind, controlled trials of calcium supplementation during pregnancy. On the basis of the results of the five randomized, controlled trials available, the risk of high blood pressure was lower in women with low baseline dietary calcium (900 mg. intake per day). These results show that calcium supplementation during pregnancy for women with deficient calcium intake is a promising preventive strategy. (Villar)

In a study at the University of Florida Health Science Center in Jacksonville, researchers found that 2,000 mg. of calcium a day reduced the onset of high blood pressure in pregnant women by 54%.

Muscles and Nerves

Calcium deficiency increases risk for muscle cramps and restless-legs syndrome. Giving a mineral supplement with high amounts of calcium to growing children who are experiencing leg pain can quickly bring relief to them.

Calcium is vitally important when it comes to properly functioning muscles. Contraction and relaxation of muscle tissues depends on the presence of calcium. Calcium ions inside our cells move from one spot to another very quickly. This changes the electrical charge of certain proteins in the muscle cell so that the proteins change shape. These proteins tighten up and, in effect, pass along the tightening action to increase the tension.

As proteins shorten the muscle cells, the muscle contracts. When the calcium ions move back to their former positions, the proteins ratchet down from their state of peak tension, and the muscle relaxes. If you have too little calcium in your cells, however, the muscle cells tend to stay in the tightened position and you'll become more prone to muscle cramps.

Along with other electrically aggressive minerals like potassium, calcium also allows our nerves to transmit messages. Because the electrically charged calcium ions in cells rapidly shift position, an electrical charge is handed along the chain of nerve cells. The result is that a small electrical current travels along the nerve. Once the current reaches the end of the nerve, it triggers the release of a neurotransmitter, a chemical that allows the message to be relayed to another cell.

In the heart, calcium's role in both muscle contraction and nerve transmission comes into play. Calcium continually interacts with potassium and sodium in a carefully orchestrated sequence to produce a heartbeat. You would have to be seriously ill to be so low on calcium that it affects your heart, but it does happen. Doctors sometimes use drugs called calcium channel blockers to slow down and regulate heartbeat in people with high blood pressure. These drugs temper the shift of calcium in and out of cells.

Note: If you are experiencing muscle cramps and are supplementing only calcium and not receiving relief, be sure to try a broad spectrum mineral supplement high in not only calcium, but also magnesium and potassium.

Cancer

Cancer is associated with anaerobic (deficiency of oxygen) conditions, resulting in the fermentation of glucose into lactic acid causing a marked drop in cellular pH. As a buffering agent, calcium (if available in the body in adequate amounts) can reduce acidity by increasing the pH of a cell from 7.4 to 8.5. In this environment, cancer cells die (while healthy cells thrive) as they cannot survive in an environment outside the range of 6.6-7.4. Thus, healthy, slightly alkaline cell conditions do not allow cancerous cells to exist.

Testing Your pH

It is easy to test the pH of your saliva, which is a reflection of the pH of your blood and cells. pH paper (with a range of 4.5 to 7.5) can be purchased at most pharmacies. Do not put anything into your mouth for at least two hours before pH is tested, as it will alter the results. Swallow a few times before placing the paper in your mouth to do the test. Your results indicate:

7.5 *(to 8.5) (dark blue) – healthy, slightly basic*

6.5 *(blue-green) – weakly acidic*

Cancer patients are usually around **4.5** *(bright yellow) indicating acidity.*

Colon Cancer

Calcium may also play a role in preventing colon cancer. Calcium in the colon acts as a protective agent by binding with cancer-promoting agents such as fatty acids and bile acids, the digestive fluids secreted by the liver. The toxic effects are neutralized and they are excreted more rapidly, along with intestinal cells that might be cancer generators. This protects the epithelial lining of the intestinal tract. (Lipkin)

Calcium also helps to prevent the absorption of toxic minerals such as lead by interfering with cellular transport. Unfortunately, it can interfere with minerals that we may need more of, such as iron, zinc, copper and manganese. That's why calcium supplements are recommended at mealtime (and not after meals when fiber supplements are recommended).

Breast Cancer

Decreased calcium and Vitamin D intake and high dietary fat are associated with breast cancer. Decreased dietary calcium and Vitamin D in a high-fat diet induce adverse changes in the mammary gland and several other organs, which can be reversed by increasing dietary calcium and Vitamin D. This suggests a possible role for increased dietary calcium and Vitamin D in the chemoprevention of these cancers. (Lipkin)

Insomnia

Calcium is essential for the nervous system. A minor deficiency often causes insomnia as calcium is needed to release the amino acid tryptophan which is involved in the synthesis of the sleep hormone, melatonin. (Gasser)

Sleep studies show that there is a relationship between sleep, calcium and parathyroid hormone (PTH). Total plasma calcium was significantly related to cycles of rapid eye movement sleep and to cycles of stage 2 sleep. PTH and calcium were significantly interrelated. PTH and calcium were more closely related to sleep stages than to each other. These results suggest that the regulation of PTH and calcium is complex and may involve interactions with the nervous system. (Kripke)

Premenstrual Cramps

A recent study shows that 1,200 mg. elemental calcium in the form of calcium carbonate reduces premenstrual symptoms, including mood swings, food cravings, pain or tenderness and bloating. The study also illustrates a relationship between PMS and calcium deficiency.

Susan Thys-Jacobs, the head researcher in the calcium project and endocrinologist at St. Luke's-Roosevelt Hospital Center in New York, describes PMS as "the clinical manifestation of functional hypocalcemia and secondary hyperparathyroidsm," a situation that occurs due to calcium deficiency. Thys-Jacobs became interested in a calcium-PMS connection when she noticed that many premenstrual symptoms, including muscle tension, irritability and pain, are shared by hypocalcemic patients whose condition is caused by clinically low calcium levels. Her 1995 pilot showed that calcium levels in test subjects with PMS were below the norm. In addition, levels of two other substances, 25-hydroxyvitamin D and parathyroid hormone, were also low, causing the parathyroid gland to malfunction and send the body false signals about its calcium levels. As a result, the body can't regulate calcium efficiently.

By the third month of the study, almost half of the women taking calcium reported less irritability, depression and food cravings. The placebo group consistently reported inferior results in symptom reduction. Only a little more than a quarter of the placebo group felt better by the third month, and a third had less food craving. Breast pain and joint tenderness were significantly improved with calcium supplementation: While a little over half of the calcium group had less breast pain and joint tenderness, the entire placebo group reported more physical discomfort in these areas. (Thys-Jacobs)

Kidney Stones

For years people have believed that calcium supplementation can increase risk of kidney stones. In reality, calcium supplementation may help prevent them! Studies show that the risk of kidney stone disease **decreases** rather than increases among individuals who had a higher calcium intake. (Curhan, Domrongkitchaiporn)

Dietary modification may play an important role in reducing the likelihood of stone recurrence. Notably, dietary calcium restriction should be avoided only in individuals who have had a calcium oxalate kidney stone. (Curhan)

Calcium Sources

Consuming calcium with foods containing calcium co-factors aids calcium absorption. (This is why Vitamin D is added to milk products.) Tofu is a pretty good calcium source, and fortified soy drinks usually provide as much calcium as milk. Cooking greens in the cabbage family (kale, collards, mustard greens, turnip greens) have as much calcium as milk, and unlike the calcium in spinach, it is just as absorbable. But, statistics show that few people get enough calcium from foods. Fortunately, supplements are equally good sources—especially when taken with or just after meals, to enhance absorption and utilization.

What you need to know about supplements

Calcium comes in many different supplemental forms. The "elemental calcium" listing on the label will tell you how much calcium it contains. If the label does not indicate how much elemental calcium is in each tablet, you can use the table below. If you're taking a 500 mg. tablet of calcium carbonate, for example, it contains 40% elemental calcium (200 mgs. of calcium from each tablet). Here are the typical percentages of actual calcium in supplement products.

Supplement	Elemental Calcium (%)
Calcium carbonate	40
Dicalcium phosphate	38
Bone meal	31
Hydroxyapatite	30
Oyster shell	28
Dolomite	22
Calcium citrate	21
Calcium lactate	13
Calcium gluconate	9

NOTE: *This is **not** an indication of the quality of the supplement - it merely shows the level of calcium they contain.*

Calcium carbonate and other insoluble forms (dolomite, bone meal and oyster shell) are the cheapest sources. Calcium carbonate may seem to be the most concentrated form, however, it is very difficult to absorb. Calcium tablets must be dissolved by stomach acid and ionized before it can be absorbed. Studies in post-menopausal women suggest that about 40% are so deficient in stomach acid that they can absorb only about 20% as much calcium from calcium carbonate as persons with normal stomach acid. In addition, dolomite, bone meal and unrefined calcium carbonate can be unacceptably high in lead.

Calcium chelates (lactate, aspartate, gluconate, orotate, hydroxyapatite, fossilized coral) are already soluble and ionized, and therefore **better absorbed** than insoluble forms, especially by persons with low stomach acid. Chelates also tend to contain less lead than the insoluble forms. Soluble calcium chelates usually do cost more, and you'll usually need two pills to deliver the 500-600 mg. elemental calcium typically found in one tablet or capsule of calcium carbonate.

Does your calcium tablet dissolve?

Your calcium tablet should dissolve in a glass of vinegar at room temperature. (Vinegar has a similar pH as our stomach acid.) Stir it around a few times and after 30 minutes the tablet should dissolve into fine particles.

You do not absorb all of the elemental calcium contained in a tablet – only about 30%.

Calcium carbonate is probably the most difficult to absorb by the body. Calcium citrate-malate is one of the best-absorbed.

If not, the tablets would probably have a hard time dissolving in your stomach and are pretty much useless.

In a similar test of 21 commercial calcium products, 11 brands failed this test. (Shangraw) When shopping for a good calcium/mineral supplement, don't let marketing hype and price convince you. The least expensive brand certainly cannot be the best buy if you do not assimilate any of the calcium, and the most expensive brand may just be an attempt to entice you to pay for a lot of misleading advertising claims.

Calcium Side Effects

According to the National Institute of Health, it should be safe for adults to consume up to 2,000 mg. of calcium every day without adverse side effects. An intake over 2,000 may lower the absorption of certain medications, such as tetracycline, and of some nutrients, including iron. Overuse of calcium carbonate (for example, which is the active ingredient in Tums® and other antacids) can also lead to severe kidney damage and other problems related to calcium toxicity. While non-chelated calcium (like calcium carbonate and calcium salts) can quickly neutralize gastric acids, if used for extended periods, it can cause acid rebound. In the elderly especially, these forms of calcium can cause gastric irritation, constipation, diarrhea, flatulence, nausea and bloating.

Effects due to the excess intake of calcium can be reduced by dividing your daily dose into two or three smaller doses.

Calcium citrate, lactate or gluconate can be taken between meals without absorption problems, and won't interfere with absorption of iron and other trace minerals. All other forms of supplemental calcium are best absorbed when taken with food. Avoid taking mineral supplements at the same time as large amounts of fiber (or the fiber will carry the calcium out of the body before it can be absorbed (in the intestinal tract). To further aid absorption, get 400 IU of Vitamin D daily from sunlight, fortified foods or supplements. It is not necessary to take them together.

Foods High in Calcium

Dairy products, tofu, fish, eggs, cereal products, nuts, seeds, beans, soy, soy products, figs and vegetables (especially green leafy) are high in calcium. Meat contains some calcium, but like dairy products, is not a good source to rely upon because its protein and phosphorus content actually contribute to calcium excretion. "Calcium fortified" foods are abundant and can be found in breakfast cereals, soup, orange juice, etc.

The degree of calcium absorption from different foods varies greatly. Vegetables such as broccoli, brussels sprouts, Chinese cabbage (bok choy), green cabbage, cauliflower, kale and kohlrabi contain a much higher rate of calcium the body can use (averaging 55-60% absorption compared to only 32% for most dairy products.) Tofu and dairy products are similar in calcium content and absorption. (See the chart on page 34.)

Food Source	**Calcium** (approx.)
Seaweed (Wakame) - 3.5 oz., dry	960 mg.
Seaweed (Nori) - 3.5 oz., dry	420 mg.
Low fat yogurt (plain) -1 cup	420 mg.
Sesame seeds (unhulled) -1 Tbsp.	381 mg.
Low fat yogurt (fruit flavored) -1 cup	350 mg.
Sardines (canned) - 3 oz.	372 mg.
Garbanzo beans (chick peas) -1 cup	300 mg.
Skim milk -1 cup	300 mg.
Calcium fortified orange juice - 8 oz.	300 mg.
Calcium fortified cereal -1 cup	300 mg.
Figs -10 dried	270 mg.
Salmon (canned with bones) - 3.5 oz.	259 mg.
Tofu (processed with calcium) - 4 oz.	250 mg.
Cheese (cheddar, colby, swiss, etc.) -1 oz.	220 mg.
Mackerel - 3 oz. canned	200 mg.
Broccoli (cooked) -1 cup	178 mg.
Broccoli (raw) - 1.5 cups (7 oz.)	206 mg.
Greens (turnip, collard, mustard) -1/2 cup	120-170 mg.
Almonds -1/2 cup	160 mg.
Hazelnuts -1/2 cup	140 mg.
Blackstrap molasses -1 Tbsp.	140 mg.
Soybeans (cooked) -1 cup	130 mg.
Spinach - 4 oz.	111 mg.
Shrimp -1 cup	80 mg.
Brown rice (cooked) - 1 cup	64 mg.
Orange -1 medium	60 mg.
Corn tortilla -1 medium	60 mg.
Peanuts -1/2 cup	60 mg.

Food	Serving Size	Calcium Content (mg.)	Fractional Absorption (%)
Cow's milk	1 cup	300	32
Almonds, dry roasted	1 oz.	80	21
Almond butter	1 Tbsp.	43	21
Beans,			
Red	1 cup	90	17
Great northern/navy	1 cup	121-128	17
White/pinto	1 cup	161-200	17
Broccoli, boiled	**1 cup**	**178**	**53**
Brussels sprouts, boiled	**1 cup**	**56**	**64**
Chinese cabbage (bok choy), boiled	**1 cup**	**158**	**54**
Cabbage, green, boiled	**1 cup**	**50**	**65**
Cauliflower, boiled	**1 cup**	**34**	**69**
Kale, boiled	**1 cup**	**94**	**59**
Kohlrabi, boiled	**1 cup**	**40**	**67**
Sesame seeds, hulled	1 oz.	37	21
Sesame seeds, unhulled	1 oz.	381	21
Sesame seed butter (tahini)	1 Tbsp.	64	21
Soymilk, Semblence	1 cup	200	31
Soymilk, Edensoy	1 cup	95	31
Soymilk, Vitasoy	1 cup	76	31
Spinach, boiled	1 cup	244	5.1
Tofu, firm	1/2 cup	258	32
Tofu, med.	1/2 cup	130	32
Turnip greens, boiled	**1 cup**	**198**	**52**

Total calcium content per serving. *This gives the calcium content in mg. of calcium per serving. Source: Pennington's Food Values of Portions Commonly Used, 1989.*

Fractional absorption. *This tells us how much calcium will be absorbed from a food. derived from Connie Weaver's work at Purdue University in the U.S.*

Fossilized Coral Calcium

Fossilized coral calcium was first discovered in 1979 when a British journalist from the *Guinness Book of Records* was sent to Okinawa to interview the world's oldest documented living person who, at the time, was an energetic 115-year-old in remarkably good health. His health and vitality was that of a person half his age.

Much of the Okinawa population is elderly, seldom dying before the age of 95, and enjoy remarkable health. Arthritis, heart disease, cancer and other debilitating diseases are practically nonexistent. A team of researchers found that neither the climate nor the diet of Okinawa was their secret, but the secret was in the water, which contained large deposits of minerals from fossilized stony coral. The island of Okinawa is built up from fossilized coral. When it rains, it erodes the reefs, producing mineral-rich water which they called, "milk of the ocean." They drink large quantities of this daily. Because of this their mineral intake is very high. It is estimated that their daily intake of calcium is 70 times the Daily Value (DV), 22 times the DV of magnesium, 18 times the DV of potassium, 120 times the DV of fluoride, etc.

Interestingly, other cultures who are well known for their longevity, the Tibetians, Hunzas, Titicacas in Puru, are societies living in mountainous regions. Their water, containing glacial-crushed minerals is also often milky white in color and is known as the "milk of the mountains."

Stony coral (hermatype) forms its shell or skeleton from the minerals in the sea, mainly calcium, magnesium, sulfur, silicon and around 70 others. For this reason, coral sand or granulated coral, which consists of the fossilized skeletons of stony coral, is made up of approximately 90% of calcium carbonate (chelated) and abundant amounts of many other minerals that are necessary to maintain health.

Fossilized stony coral is used as a food supplement made from coral sand that provides calcium, magnesium, sulfur, silicon and almost 70 other minerals. Fossilized stony coral has a much better absorption rate than many other calcium supplements do because of several reasons described on the next page.

Fossilized coral grains are from the skeletal structure of reef-building coral that are no longer living. Coral miners are not allowed to disturb the living reefs, which are the nursery grounds and habitat of many fishes, invertebrates and plants. The methods use in harvesting does not and will not destroy living coral reefs or in any way damage the environment, but helps to offer needed nutrients for our good health.

Acid/Alkaline Maintenance

Optimum alkalinity at the cellular level equates to optimum health. Scientists have long known that the maintenance of body fluids (such as blood and saliva) at a slightly alkaline pH of 7.1 to 7.5 is critical to cellular health. Degenerative conditions (especially cancerous cells) live and proliferate in an acidic environment (a pH below 7). By adding one gram (about 1/4 teaspoon) of fossilized coral to drinking water (distilled is best) the pH is raised to an alkaline level between 9.5 and 11.5. Drinking this helps maintain a healthy pH in the body.

Bioavailability

The form of calcium in fossilized coral is quickly

bioavailable to the body. It is naturally chelated, meaning the mineral is bound to a carrier molecule (largely carbonic acid) which allows the calcium (and other minerals) from the ocean to be readily absorbed and bioavailable to the cells.

Coral calcium lowers the surface tension of the water, allowing it to penetrate and hydrate the cells easily, carrying in nutrients and removing the toxins and waste residue.

In order for ordinary calcium (and all minerals) to do its work, the body must convert it to an ionic form or the calcium is not efficiently utilized.

Because of the shape of the mineral crystals in fossilized coral, it is more bioavailable than other mineral sources. Most calcium carbonate crystals have a square or hexagon shape, but years of erosion breaks down and modifies the shape in fossilized coral to a more circular rhombus (Aragonite). This special shape is six times more soluble in water than regular calcium carbonate!

The larger solubility means that it has a higher degree of electronic dissociation or ionization potential. When an acid, base (alkali) or salt is dissociated in water or other solvent, a part or all of the molecules are broken into parts called ions of which some are charged with positive (cations) or negative (anions) energy. This is required for minerals to effectively biologically react in the body.

Minerals: It's *Not* Just About Calcium

Minerals are defined as naturally-occurring inorganic substances from non-biologic origin found in the earth, sea water or the human body.

Calcium makes up 35% of the body's minerals. It is scientifically documented that more than 150 diseases are related to calcium deficiency. However, it does not work alone. In nature, it is not found alone, as it is not alone in the body where there are over 70 different minerals.

Phosphorus is the second most abundant mineral in the body. It functions with Vitamin D and calcium and is found in every cell in the body. It is essential for energy production, muscle contraction, digestion and the pH balance of the blood.

Phosphorus deficiencies are extremely rare as it is very available so in many foods eaten today. Food sources include meat, fish, poultry, eggs, beans, whole grains, nuts and seeds. Phosphoric acid, which is contained in soda pop, is also a major source of phosphorus for pop drinkers. Unlike calcium, which is difficult for the body to absorb, phosphorus is easy for the body to absorb. Too much phosphorus can actually cause calcium/bone loss. This is common in individuals who consume a diet high in animal protein.

Magnesium is an essential mineral found inside all cells where it is involved in many metabolic processes. The functions of magnesium include enzyme reactions, energy release (ATP), neuromuscular contraction, calcium absorption, protein synthesis and body temperature regulation. It also helps utilization of Vitamins C and E and the B Complex. Because magnesium is very alkaline, it helps regulate the acid-alkaline balance of the body.

Some experts believe that a calcium deficiency is actually caused by a magnesium deficiency which requires magnesium supplementation. Magnesium, like

ELEMENTAL ANALYSIS OF FOSSILIZED CORAL

Elements	Result (ppm)	Elements	Result (ppm)
Aluminum	180	Molybdenum	<0.08
Antimony	0.37	Neodymium	1.11
Arsenic	0.38	Nickel	<0.08
Barium	2.29	Niobium	<0.09
Beryllium	<0.06	Nitrogen	<0.005
Bismuth	<0.09	Osmium	<0.2
Bromine	0.14	Palladium	<0.025
Boron	0.182	Phosphorus	94.1
Cadmium	<0.1	Platinum	<0.03
Calcium	391,000	Potassium	32.5
Carbon	119,000	Praseodymium	2.73
Chlorine	275	Rhenium	<0.2
Chromium	0.625	Rhodium	<0.02
Cobalt	0.091	Rubidium	0.22
Copper	<0.2	Ruthenium	0.081
Deuterium*	150	Samarium	<0.05
Dysprosium	0.18	Scandium	0.049
Erbium	5.19	Selenium	<0.08
Europium	<0.1	Silicon	1,280
Fluorine	0.67	Silver	0.38
Gadolinium	0.094	Sodium	129
Gallium	0.692	Strontium	295
Germanium	0.191	Sulfur	1,780
Gold	<0.05	Tantalum	<0.1
Hafnium	<0.15	Tellurium	<0.2
Holmium	0.091	Terbium	0.091
Hydrogen	1,100	Thallium	1.24
Indium	<0.06	Thorium	0.101
Iodine	1.22	Thulium	0.052
Iridium	<0.04	Tin	0.198
Iron	510	Titanium	5.88
Lanthanum	0.323	Tungsten	<0.09
Lead	<0.08	Vanadium	0.267
Lithium	0.66	Ytterbium	0.051
Lutetium	0.078	Yttrium	0.461
Magnesium	4,190	Zinc	2.51
Manganese	26.9	Zirconium	<0.08
Mercury	<0.01		

* Isotope of Hydrogen

Halstead, BW; *Fossil Stony Coral Minerals and Their Nutritional Application.* A World Life Research Institute Publication. Cannon Beach, OR 1999, pg 25.

a key, opens the door for calcium to be absorbed by bone. It allows us to use our body's calcium supply more efficiently. Without magnesium, calcium builds up in soft tissues where it doesn't belong and cannot be incorporated into bone properly. Magnesium favors the hormonal mechanism that puts calcium back into bones.

In one study, volunteers on magnesium-depleted diets, who were given calcium supplements, became deficient in calcium. When the subjects were given magnesium, their calcium levels rose within a few days. Calcium must have adequate magnesium to work.

Food sources of magnesium include nuts and seeds, fresh green vegetables, soybeans, beans, peas, unprocessed whole grains (especially barley and wheat), seafood, figs, chocolate, corn and apples. Meat, milk and dairy products are **poor** sources of magnesium.

Manganese is vital to the development of bones, ligaments, nerves and also is important to proper digestion. It is also important in sex hormone and milk production and functions as a catalyst and enzyme activator. Recent studies show a manganese deficiency contributes to excess blood sugar.

Manganese is found in whole-grain cereals, egg yolks, nuts, seeds and green vegetables. **NOTE:** A great deal of manganese is lost in the processing of foods.

Zinc is essential for proper bone maintenance. Bone tissue contains about 200 mcg. per gram of zinc. Several studies report that the average American diet only provides only 46-63% of the DV for zinc.

Sulfur is the third most abundant mineral in the body and the fourth most abundant mineral in fossilized coral. It is involved in the synthesis of all connective tissue (especially skin, joints, etc.) in the body. It is also needed to produce insulin and is an important detoxifier in the body.

Silicon is an important component for collagen, bones, in arterial metabolism and in the prevention of arthritis and osteoporosis.

Iron plays a central role in the heme molecule in red blood cells. This molecule is responsible for oxygen transport.

Strontium is believed to be important for strong healthy bones and tooth structure.

Copper is needed for bone development and mineralization and for hemoglobin function. It is also critical for healthy joints. About 19% of the body's copper is found in bone tissue.

Fluoride and **sodium** are among the many trace elements necessary for mineralization. These minerals act as "mortar" giving bone hardness, strength and rigidity.

Silica and sulfur are also very important components of healthy bone.

	In Coral Calcium	*In the Body*
Calcium	391,000 ppm	14,000 ppm
Magnesium	4,190 ppm	270 ppm
Sulfur	1,780 ppm	2,000 ppm
Silicon	1,280 ppm	260 ppm
Iron	510 ppm	60 ppm
Strontium	295 ppm	NA

For more information on fossilized coral, Bruce Halstead, MD, has written an extensive book, Fossil Stony Coral Minerals and their Nutritional Application, Health Digest Publishing Company, P.O. Box 1100, Cannon Beach, OR 97110. E-mail: Info@coralminerals.com

Bibliography

Aerssens J; Declerck K; Maeyaert B; Boonen S; Dequeker J; The effect of modifying dietary calcium intake pattern on the circadian rhythm of bone resorption. Arthritis and Metabolic Bone Disease Research Unit, K.U. Leuven, U.Z. Pellenberg, Weligerveld Pellenberg, Belgium.Calcif Tissue Int 1999 Jul;65(1):34-40.

Allen SH "Primary osteoporosis. Methods to combat bone loss that accompanies aging." *Postgrad Med* 1993 Jun;93(8):43-6, 49-50, 53-5.

Aloia, J.K., *Metabolism*, 1990: 39: 35-38.

American Journal of Clinical Nutrition, 1982; 35;1048-1075.

Appleton, Nancy, "Healthy Bones" Avery Publishing, Garden City Park, NY,1991.

Baeksgaard L, Andersen KP, Hyldstrup L; Calcium and vitamin D supplementation increases spinal BMD in healthy, postmenopausal women. Osteoporos Int. 1998;8(3):255-60.

Barger-Lux MJ; Heaney RP; The role of calcium intake in preventing bone fragility, hypertension, and certain cancers. J Nutr 1994 Aug;124(8 Suppl):1406S-1411S.

Benke, P.J.; et al; "Osteoporotic bone disease in the pyridoxine deficient rat" *Biochem Med* 1972, 6: 526-535.

Bucher HC, Cook RJ, Guyatt GH, et al.; Effects of dietary calcium supplementation on blood pressure Ca meta-analysis of randomized controlled trials. JAMA 1996;275:1016-22.

Brazier, M., Fardelonne, P., Bollony, R., Sebert, J.L., Desmet,G.; *Euro. J. Drug Metab Pharmacokinet* 1991, Spec No 3, pg 161-165.

Brenton, D.P and Dent, C.E.; "Ideopathic Juvenile Osteoporosis" *Inborn Errors of Metabolism* Ed. Bickel, H. & Stern J. Publ. MTP Press Limited 1976 pg 222-239.

Chestnut CH; "Do we have any alternative to sex steroids in the prevention and treatment of osteoporosis?" *Baillieres Clin Obstet Gynaecol* 1991 Dec;5(4):857-65.

Christianson, D., et al; *Eur. J. Clin. Invest.* 1981;11: 305-308.

Curhan GC; Dietary calcium, dietary protein, and kidney stone formation. Channing Laboratory, Department of Medicine, Brigham and Women's Hospital, Boston, Mass. Miner Electrolyte Metab 1997;23(3-6):261-4.

Davies, I.J.T.; Osteogenesis Imperfecta Treated with Microcrystalline Hydroxyapatite Compound" Osteoporosis, A Multi-disciplinary Problem Ed Dixon. (1983) Royal Society of Medicine International Congress and symposium Series No. 55 Public Academic Press Inc. (London) and Royal Society of Medicine pg, 279-286.

Dawson-Hughes B; Dallal GE; Krall EA; Sadowski L; Sahyoun N; Tannenbaum S A controlled trial of the effect of calcium supplementation on bone density in postmenopausal women. *N Engl J Med* 1990 Sep 27;323(13):878-83.

Dent, C.E., Davies, I.J.T.; Calcium metabolism in bone disease; effects of treatment with microcrystalline calcium hydroxyapatite compound with dihydrotachysterol. Journal of the Royal Society of Medicine, (1980) 73;780-787.

Dodds, R.A. et al; "Abnormalities in fracture healing induced by vitamin B-6 deficiency in rats" Bone 1986, 7; 489-495.

Domrongkitchaiporn S; et al; Risk of calcium oxalate nephrolithiasis after calcium or combined calcium and calcitriol supplementation in postmenopausal women. Osteoporos Int 2000;11(6):486-92.

Dyckner T, Wester PO. Effect of magnesium on blood pressure. BMJ 1983;286:1847-9.

Epstein O; Kato Y; Dick R; Sherlock S "Vitamin D, hydroxyapatite, and calcium gluconate in treatment of cortical bone thinning in postmenopausal women with primary biliary cirrhosis." Am J Clin Nutr 1982 Sep;36(3):426-30.

Eriksson SA; Lindgren JU "Combined treatment with calcitonin and 1,25-dihydroxyvitamin D3 for osteoporosis in women." Calcif Tissue Int 1993 Jul; 53(1): 26-8.

Evans, Gary, "There are Two C's in Osteoporosis" Bemidji State University, Bemidji, MN.

Gambacciani M; Spinetti A; et al. "Prospective evaluation of calcium and estrogen administration on bone mass and metabolism after ovariectomy." *Gynecol Endocrinol* 1995 Jun;9(2):131-5.

Gasser PJ; Gern WARegulation of melatonin synthesis in rainbow trout (Oncorhyncus mykiss) pineal organs: effects of calcium depletion and calcium channel drugs. Gen Comp Endocrinol 1997 Feb;105(2):210-7.

Goyer RA; Epstein S; Bhattacharyya M; Korach KS; Pounds J "Environmental risk factors for osteoporosis *Environ Health Perspect* 1994 Apr;102(4):390-4.

Halpern GM; Van de Water J; Delabroise AM; Keen CL; Gershwin ME "Comparative uptake of calcium from milk and a calcium-rich mineral water in lactose intolerant adults: implications for treatment of osteoporosis." *Am J Prev Med* 1991 Nov-Dec;7(6):379-83.

Halstead, BW; Fossil Stony Coral Minerals and Their Nutritional Application. A World Life Research Institute Publication. Cannon Beach, OR 1999.

Hasling C; Charles P; Jensen FT; Mosekilde L "A comparison of the effects of oestrogen/progestogen, high-dose oral calcium, intermittent cyclic etidronate and an ADFR regime on calcium kinetics and bone mass in postmenopausal women with spinal osteoporosis." *Osteoporos Int* 1994 Jul;4(4):191-203.

Hayashi K, Uenoyama K, Matsuguchi N. et al; The affinity of bone to hydroxyapatite and alumina in experimentally induced osteoporosis. J Arthroplasty 1989 Sep;4(3):257-62.

Hollo, I., et al., "Osteopenia" Ann Intern Med, 1977; 86: 637.

Johnson, C.C., et. al.,"Changes in skeletal tissue during the aging process" Nutrition Reviews, 1992;50, no.2, pg 385-387.

Kariya, Y., Watabe S. et al, J. Biol. Chem (US) 1990 265 (9);pg5081-5.

Kawano Y; Yoshimi H; Matsuoka H; et al; Calcium supplementation in patients with essential hypertension: assessment by office, home and ambulatory blood pressure. J Hypertens 1998 Nov;16(11):1693-9.

Khadzhiev A, Rachev E, Katsarova M, Cherveniashki S; The results of a clinical trial of the preparation Ossopan. Akush Ginekol (Sofiia) 1990;29(4):85-7.

Kohara N; Clinical study of concerning factors of decreased bone mineral content in hemodialysis patients. Nippon Jinzo Gakkai Shi 1991 Jun;33(6):587-96.

Kripke DF; Lavie P; Parker D; Huey L; Deftos LJ; Plasma parathyroid hormone and calcium are related to sleep stage cycles. J Clin Endocrinol Metab 1978 Nov;47(5):1021-7.

Kveton JF; Friedman CD; Piepmeier JM; Costantino PD "Reconstruction of suboccipital craniectomy defects with hydroxyapatite cement: a preliminary report." Laryngoscope 1995 Feb;105(2):156-9.

Landman JO; Schweitzer DH; Frolich M; Hamdy NA; Papapoulos SE "Recovery of serum calcium concentrations following acute hypocalcemia in patients with osteoporosis on long-term oral therapy with the bisphosphonate pamidronate. J Clin Endocrinol Metab 1995 Feb;80(2):524-8.

Lipkin M; Newmark HL; Vitamin D, calcium and prevention of colorectal cancer: a review. Weill Medical College of Cornell University, J Am Coll Nutr 1999 Oct;18(5 Suppl):392S-397S.

Lipkin M; et al; Cyclogenase-2 over expression and tumor formation are blocked by sunlindac in murine model of familial adenomatous polyposis. Cacner Res. 56;2556-2560.

Marsh AG; Sanchez TV; Midkelsen O; Keiser J; Mayor G "Cortical bone density of adult lacto-ovo-vegetarian and omnivorous women." J Am Diet Assoc 1980 Feb;76(2):148-51.

McCarron DA; Calcium metabolism in hypertension. Division of Nephrology, Hypertension and Clinical Pharmacology, Oregon Health Sciences University, Portland Keio J Med 1995 Dec;44(4):105-14.

Mills, T.J., Davis, H. Broadhurst, B.W.; The Use of Whole Bone in the Treatment of Fracture's. Manitoba Medical Review, 1965;45:92-96.

Metz JA; Anderson JJ; Gallagher PN Jr; "Intakes of calcium, phosphorus, and protein, and physical-activity level are related to radial bone mass in young adult women" Am J Clin Nutr 1993 Oct;58(4):537-42.

Mongiorgi R, Krajewski A "Mineralogical alterations in osteoporotic bone tissue structure." Biomaterials 1981 Jul;2(3):147-50.

Motoyama T, Sano H, Fukuzaki H, et al. Oral magnesium supplementation in patients with essential hypertension. Hypertension 1989;13:227-32.

Nawata H; Tanaka S; Tanaka S; et al "Aromatase in bone cell: association with osteoporosis in postmenopausal women." J Steroid Biochem Mol Biol 1995 Jun;53(1-6):165-74.

Neilson, F.H. "Effect of Dietary Boron on Mineral, Estrogen and Testosterone Metabolism in Postmenopausal Women" FASEB J 1987;1; 394-297.

Nilsen KH; Jayson MI; Dixon AS "Microcrystalline calcium hydroxyapatite compound in corticosteroid-treated rheumatoid patients: a controlled study." Br Med J 1978 Oct 21;2(6145):1124.

Ortega RM; Requejo AM; et al; Implication of calcium deficiency in the progress of periodontal diseases and osteoporosis. Departamento de Nutricion, Facultad de Farmacia, Universidad Complutense, Madrid. Nutr Hosp 1998 Nov-Dec;13(6):316-9.

Orwoll, E.S., et al "The effects of dietary protein insufficiency and excess on skeletal health" Bone 1992; 13;343-350.

Ott, S.M. et al Ann. Internal Medicine, 1989;110;267-274.

Parsons, B., Mitchell, C., Emond, A. Darby, A.J., "The Use of Sodium Fluoride and Calcium Supplements and Vitamin D in the Treatment of Axial Osteoporosis." "Osteoporosis, A Multi-disciplinary Problem" Ed Dixon. (1983) Royal Society of Medicine International Congress and symposium Series No. 55 Public Academic Press Inc. (London) and Royal Society of Medicine pg, 259-264.

Peacock M; Liu G; Carey M; et al; Effect of calcium or 25OH vitamin D3 dietary supplementation on bone loss at the hip in men and women over the age of 60. J Clin Endocrinol Metab 2000 Sep;85(9):3011-9. J Clin Endocrinol Metab. 2000 Sep;85(9):3009-10.

Pfeiffer, Naomi" Moderate Drinking may cut Osteoporosis" Medical Tribune, 1992; 3 July23;

Pines A; Raafat H; Lynn AH; et al; Clinical trial of microcrystalline hydroxyapatite compound ('Ossopan') in the prevention of osteoporosis due to corticosteroid therapy. Curr Med Res Opin 1984;8(10): 734-42.

Praet JP; Peretz A; Mets T; Rozenberg S; Comparative study of the intestinal absorption of three salts of calcium in young and elderly women. Geriatric Unit, Universitair Ziekenhuis St. Pieter, Brussels, Belgium. J Endocrinol Invest 1998 Apr;21(4):263-7.

Prince R; Devine A; Dick I; Criddle A; et al "The effects of calcium supplementation (milk powder or tablets) and exercise on bone density in postmenopausal women. *J Bone Miner Res* 1995 Jul;10(7):1068-75.

Prince RL; Smith M; et al; "Prevention of postmenopausal osteoporosis. A comparative study of exercise, calcium supplementation, and hormone-replacement therapy." *N Engl J Med* 1991 Oct 24;325(17):1189-95.

Remagen W; Prezmecky L "Bone augmentation with hydroxyapatite: histological findings in 55 cases." *Implant Dent* 1995 Fall;4(3):182-8.

Reynolds, T.M., "Hip fractures in patients may be vitamin B-6 deficient. Controlled study of serum pyridoxal-5'-phosphate." *Acta Orthop Scand* 1992, 63: 635-638.

Riggs, B.L., et al, " A New Option For Treating Osteoporosis" *New England Journal of Medicine*, (1990) 323:124-125.

Riggs, B.L., et al, " The Prevention and Treatment of Osteoporosis" *New England Journal of Medicine*, 1992;327 (9) 620-627.

Ringe JD, Keller A "Risk of osteoporosis in long-term heparin therapy of thromboembolic diseases in pregnancy: attempted prevention with ossein-hydroxyapatite" *Geburtshilfe Frauenheilkd* 1992 Jul;52(7):426-9.

Ritchie LD; King JC; Detary calcium and pregnancy-induced hypertension: is there a relation? Dep. of Nutritional Sciences, University of California, Berkeley. Am J Clin Nutr 2000 May;71(5 Suppl):1371S-4S.

Roepke, J.B. et al "Effect on smoking and vitamin B-6 supplementation during pregnancy on maternal vitamin B-6 status and infant birth weight" *Fed Proc* 1983, 42:1066.

Rubinacci A; Divieti P; Capponi A; Resmini G; Daverio R; Veglia F; Tessari L "Reduction in parathormone secretion after oral calcium loading in osteoporotic adults" *Endocrinol* 1992 Apr-Jun;17(2):55-65.

Ruegsegger P; Keller A; Dambacher MA "Comparison of the treatment effects of ossein-hydroxyapatite compound and calcium carbonate in osteoporotic females." *Osteoporosis Int* 1995 Jan;5(1):30-4.

Shangraw, R. "Factors to consider in the selection of a calcium supplement" Special Topic Conference on Osteoporosis. October, 1987.

Snow-Harter CM "Bone health and prevention of osteoporosis in active and athletic women." *Clin Sports Med* 1994 Apr;13(2):389-404

Spencer H; Kramer L; Osis D; Wiatrowski E; Norris C; Lender M "Effect of calcium, phosphorus, magnesium, and aluminum on fluoride metabolism in man." *Ann N Y Acad Sci* 1980;355:181-94.

Spencer H; "Effect on small doses of aluminum-containing antacids on calcium and phosphorus metabolism" *American Journal of Clinical Nutrition* 1982; 36:32-40.

Spencer H; Kramer L; et al, "Antacid-induced calcium loss" *Arch Internal Medicine* 1983;143:657-659.

Stamp, T.C.B., Jenkins, M.V. Walker, P.G., and Mitchell, T.H. " Treatment of osteoporosis and MCHC compound and sodium fluoride." "Osteoporosis, A Multi-disciplinary Problem" Ed Dixon. (1983) Royal Society of Medicine International Congress and symposium Series No. 55 Public Academic Press Inc. (London) and Royal Society of Medicine pg, 287-290.

Stellon, A., A. Davis., A Webb., and R. Williams. "Microcrystalline Hydroxy apatite compound in prevention of bone loss in corticosteriod-treated patients with chronic actice hepatitis." *Postgraduate Medicine Journal* (1985) 61, 791-796.

Stephan, J.J., Pospichal J., et al. "Prospective Trial of Ossein-Hydroxyapatite compound in surgically induced postmenopausal women." *Bone* (1989) 10, 179-185.

Stevenson JC; Hillard TC; Lees B; Whitcroft SI; Ellerington MC;

Thys-Jacobs S, Alvir M. Calcium-regulating hormones across the menstrual cycle: evidence of secondary hyperparathyroidism in women with PMS. J Clin Endocrinol Metab. 1995; 80(7): 2227-2232.

Thys-Jacobs S, Starkey, P, Bernstein D, Tain J. Calcium carbonate and the premenstrual syndrome: effects on premenstrual and menstrual symptoms. Am J Obstet Gynecol. 1998; 179(2): 444-452.

Tremollieres F; Pouilles JM; Ribot C "Effect of long-term administration of progestogen on post-menopausal bone loss: result of a two-year, controlled randomized study." *Clin Endocrinol* (Oxf) 1993 Jun;38(6):627-31.

Villar J; Belizan JM; Same nutrient, different hypotheses: disparities in trials of calcium supplementation during pregnancy. UNDP/ UNFPA/ WHO/ World Bank Special Programme of Research, Development and Research Training in Human Reproduction, World Health Organization, Geneva, Switzerland. Am J Clin Nutr 2000 May;71(5 Suppl):1375S-9S.

Walker, Alexander "Osteoporosis and Calcium Deficiency" *American Journal of Clinical Nutrition*, Vol. 16, March 1965.

Windsor AC; Misra DP; Loudon JM; Staddon GE "The effect of whole-bone extract on 47 Ca absorption in the elderly." *Age Ageing* 1973 Nov; 2(4): 230-4.

Whitehead MI "Postmenopausal bone loss: does HRT always work?" Wynn Institute for Metabolic Research, London, U.K. *Int J Fertil Menopausal Stud* 1993;38 Suppl 2:88-91.

Yamamoto, M.Y., et al *J Clin Invest*, 1984;74: 507-513.

Index

Acid .5, 9-10, 19, 24, 26, 30-31, 36-38
Acidosis 19
African-American 21
Alcohol 8, 14, 17
Alkaline Maintenance 36
Almonds 33-34
Aloia 11
Alveolar 20
American 8, 10, 18, 21, 40
American Heart Association ...10, 21
Americans 15
Assimilation 10
B Complex 38
Beans 32-34, 38, 40
Bioavailability 37
Blackstrap 33
Bone 6-8, 10-11, 13, 15-20, 29-30, 38, 40-41
Breast Cancer 6, 13, 26
Broccoli 9, 32-34
Brussels sprouts 32, 34
Cabbage 28, 32, 34
Calcium Co-factors 10
Calcium Enemies 14
Calcium Side Effects 31
Calcium Sources 28
Cancer 6, 13, 24-26, 35
Cauliflower 32, 34
Cheese 9, 33
Chelates 30
Children 9, 23
Cholecalciferol 14
Colon Cancer 6, 13, 25
Copper 25, 41
Coral 5, 30, 35-37, 39, 41
Corn 33, 40
Cramps 13, 17, 23-24, 27
Dairy 6, 9-11, 14, 32, 40
Dental Health 20
Dicalcium 29
Dolomite 29-30
Dowagers Hump 17
Fiber 8, 14, 17, 32
Figs 32-33, 40
Fluoride 35, 41
Food 9, 27, 32-34, 36, 38, 40
Fossilized Coral ..5, 30, 35-37, 39, 41
Fractures 15-18
Garbanzo beans 33
Greens 28, 33-34
Hazelnuts 33
Heart 5, 7, 10, 17, 21, 24, 35
High Blood Pressure ...5-6, 13, 21-24
Hydroxyapatite 29-30
Insomnia 13, 26
Iron 13, 25, 31, 41

Kale 28, 32, 34
Kidney Stones 11, 28
Kohlrabi 32, 34
LDL 21
Mackerel 33
Magnesium .10-13, 22, 35-36, 38, 40-41
Manganese 25, 40
Meat 5, 7, 10, 14, 19, 32, 38, 40
Men 6, 8, 13, 16, 18
Minerals ..5, 7-10, 12-13, 19-20, 23, 31, 35, 37-38, 41
Mineral Balancing 12
Muscles 7, 14, 23
National Institutes of Health 5, 31
Nerves 14, 23-24, 40
Nori 33
Osteoporosis ..5, 7, 11, 13, 15-20, 41
Peanuts 15, 33
Periodontal Disease 18, 20
Phosphoric acid 5, 38
Phosphorus ..7, 10-11, 14, 19, 32, 38
PMS 27
Postmenopausal 9, 11, 30
Pregnancy-related High Blood Pressure 13, 22
Pregnant 9, 22-23
Premenstrual Cramps 27
Protein .5, 7-8, 10-11, 14, 17, 19, 32, 38
PTH 26
Salmon 33
Seaweed 33
Sesame 33-34
Shrimp 33
Silica 41
Silicon 35-36, 41
Sleep 26
Smokers 17
Smoking 14
Soybeans 33, 40
Soymilk 34
Spinach 15, 28, 33-34
Strontium 41
Sulfur 35-36, 41
Tofu 28, 32-34
Tums 31
Vegetables 32, 40
Vegetarians 7, 10
Vinegar 8, 10, 30
Vitamin D ...6, 11, 20, 26, 28, 32, 38
Vitamin D-3 .... 9, 11, 14
Vitamin A 10-11
Vitamin C 38
Women .6, 8-9, 11, 13, 15-16, 18, 20-23, 27, 30
X-rays 16
Zinc 25, 40

45

ABOUT THE AUTHOR

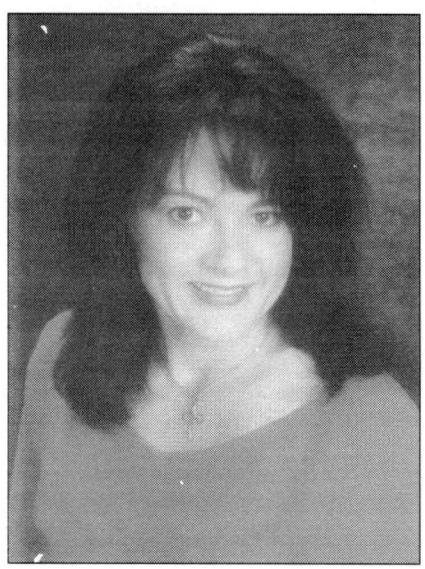

Beth M. Ley, Ph.D., has been a science writer specializing in health and nutrition for over 12 years and has written over a dozen health related books, including the best sellers, ***DHEA: Unlocking the Secrets to the Fountain of Youth*** and ***MSM: On Our Way Back to Health With Sulfur***. She wrote her own undergraduate degree program and graduated in Scientific and Technical Writing from North Dakota State University in 1987 (combination of Zoology and Journalism). Beth has her masters (1997) and doctoral degrees (1999) in Nutrition.

Beth lives in the Minnesota lakes country. She is dedicated to God and to spreading the health message. She enjoys spending time with her Dalmatians, exercises on a regular basis, eats a vegetarian, low-fat diet and takes anti-aging supplements.

Memberships: American Academy of Anti-aging, New York Academy of Sciences, Oxygen Society.

ORDER THESE GREAT BOOKS
FROM BL PUBLICATIONS!

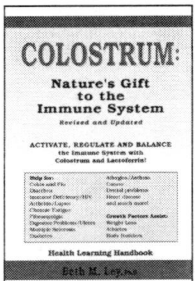

Colostrum: Nature's Gift to The Immune System
Beth M. Ley, Ph.D.,
80 pgs, $5.95

MSM: On Our Way Back To Health With Sulfur
Beth M. Ley,
40 pgs, $3.95

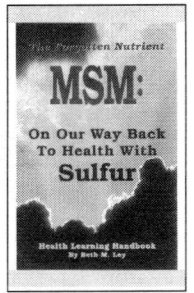

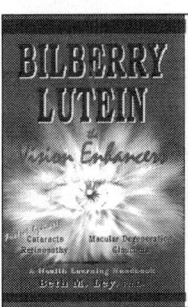

Bilberry & Lutein: The Vision Enhancers
Beth M. Ley, Ph.D.
40 pgs. $4.95

Marvelous Memory Boosters
Beth M. Ley, Ph.D.
32 pgs, $3.95

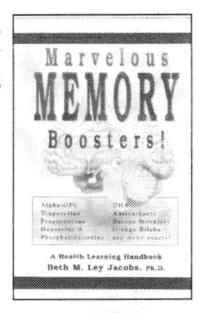

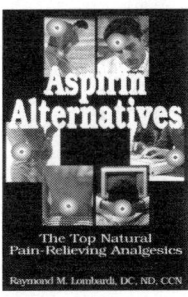

Aspirin Alternatives: The Top Natural Pain-Relieving Analgesics
Raymond Lombardi, D.C., N.D., C.C.N.,
160 pgs, $8.95

DHA: The Magnificent Marine Oil
Beth M. Ley-Jacobs, Ph.D.,
120 pgs, $6.95

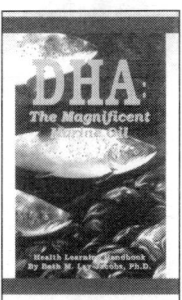

Coenzyme Q10: All Around Nutrient for All-Around Health!
Beth M. Ley-Jacobs, Ph.D.,
60 pgs, $4.95

Natural Healing Handbook
Beth M. Ley,
320 pgs. $14.95

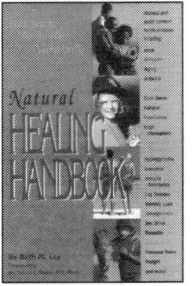

# of copies

TO PLACE AN ORDER:

___ **Aspirin Alternatives: The Top Natural Pain-Relieving Analgesics** (Lombardi) $8.95

___ **Bilberry & Lutein: The Vision Enhancers!** (Ley) $4.95

___ **Calcium: The Facts, Fossilized Coral** (Ley) $4.95

___ **Castor Oil: Its Healing Properties** (Ley) $3.95

___ **Dr. John Willard on Catalyst Altered Water** (Ley) $3.95

___ **Co Q10: All-Around Nutrient for All-Around Health** (Ley) . $4.95

___ **Colostrum: Nature's Gift to the Immune System** (Ley) $5.95

___ **DHA: The Magnificent Marine Oil** (Ley) $6.95

___ **DHEA: Unlocking the Secrets of the Fountain of Youth - 2nd Edition** (Ash & Ley) $14.95

___ **Discover the Beta Glucan Secret** (Ley) $3.95

___ **Fading: One family's journey with a women silenced by Alzheimer's** (Kraft) $12.95

___ **God Wants You Well** (Ley) $14.95

___ **Health Benefits of Probiotics** (Dash) $4.95

___ **How Did We Get So Fat? 2nd Edition** (Susser & Ley) $8.95

___ **How to Fight Osteoporosis and Win!** (Ley) $6.95

___ **Immune System Control-Colostrum & Lactoferrin** (Ley) $12.95

___ **Marvelous Memory Boosters** (Ley) $3.95

___ **Medicinal Mushrooms:** *Agaricus Blazei Murill (Ley)* $4.95

___ **MSM: On Our Way Back to Health W/ Sulfur** (Ley) $3.95

___ **Natural Healing Handbook** (Ley) $14.95

___ **Nature's Road to Recovery: Nutritional Supplements for the Alcoholic & Chemical Dependent** (Ley) $5.95

___ **PhytoNutrients: Medicinal Nutrients Found in Foods** (Ley) $3.95

___ **The Potato Antioxidant: Alpha Lipoic Acid** (Ley) $6.95

___ **Vinpocetine: Revitalize Your Brain w/ Periwinkle Extract!** (Ley) $4.95

Subtotal $ _____ Please add $4.00 for shipping. **TOTAL $** _____

Send check or money order to:
BL Publications 14325 Barnes Drive Detroit Lakes, MN 56501

Credit card orders call toll free: 1-877-BOOKS11

Also visit: www.blpbooks.com